My Smart Body:
How I Beat Endometriosis

This book is dedicated to every young girl
that has or will experience early-onset of
endometriosis.

Bavaria G.

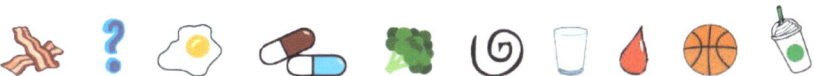

First paperback edition: August 2021

Cover Design/ Illustrations by Amanda B. Jaworski
Edited by Elizabeth A. Miles

ISBN:
ISBN:

Published by Bavaria G.
www.BavariaG.com

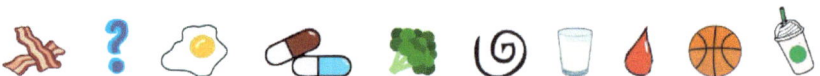

To Share or Not to Share

I really never imagined I would be able to share my story. It's the kind of conversation girls my age don't typically feel comfortable sharing. Talking about yourself is sometimes tough enough, but talking about your menstruation cycle is even more uncomfortable.

Knowing that a stranger has your story in their hands and is reading every single line, word by word, and finally learning about the pain I had to go through shakes me. Something that I was too embarrassed to tell my friends and family is now the thing I'll be telling the whole world. My mom told me that real satisfaction comes from sharing with others, but I always thought sharing would mean physical things, like a bike, a phone, even a crayon. But no, I am verbally sharing some personal details about my life with others and, might I emphasize, strangers.

And, by the way, I am only 13.

While I am a bit apprehensive and unsure how this is going to unfold, I still have the courage to share my story. I still dwell on the fact this is about my period, and it's hard to stop thinking about that. My period is hard to talk about. It's not the

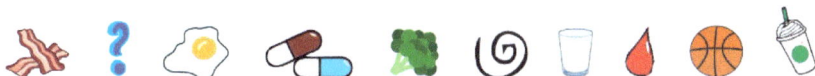

standard teenager talk, like school or basketball. I am sharing personal details about my feelings and my body, and I am literally talking about blood and how it wouldn't stop flowing for weeks.

As the adage goes, "A stitch in time saves nine." Hopefully, this can help someone from being lost and feeling helpless. I want this book to become a helping hand for someone else going through this journey with early-onset of endometriosis. I know that, for me, it felt like a long battle between me and my body. Especially in the early stages of diagnosis, when nobody quite understood what was happening, I remember how alone and scared I felt. I don't want that for anyone else. Helping others would make all of the pain seem like it was worth something. For anyone going through endometriosis, know this: Everything is going to be okay! Also, know that there are options available to help you (other than a birth control pill). I hope my story helps another girl out there because everyone deserves to be well.

Now, here's my story. Did I really say that out loud?

Ugh, I sound so corny.

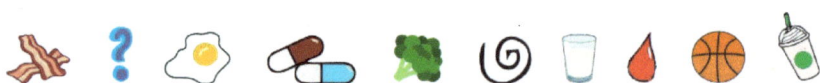

COVID

The spring of 2020 was one that nobody will ever forget. The deadly coronavirus (COVID-19) swept through the entire nation and the world, forcing everyone and everything into lockdown. All businesses, stores, schools, recreational facilities, and even some parks were closed.

Beyond the forced quarantine, COVID-19 impacted things like when I woke up in the morning, the foods I ate, when I ate, my activity level, and even my social life. Honestly, though, my social life wasn't really a big circle of people. At twelve years old, my social life consisted of a circle of a few friends I'd talk to in order to stay away from everybody else. My friends had other friends, and that did expand my circle a little bit, which was nice (sometimes).

Up until that point, I played basketball. That had been a big part of my life and helped me stay fit and healthy. But the basketball season was over thanks to COVID. Even though my friend circle had multiplied a bit, keeping in touch with everyone was a struggle. We couldn't really hang out due to the lockdown. Even conversations through text or phone calls were a struggle. At school, our teachers drank coffee, getting through the day with caffeine.

As students, our caffeine was drama. That drama was like our coffee and, as preteens, it can be hard to live without.

So, when COVID hit, everything was gone. No basketball. No going anywhere other than the grocery store. And nothing really to talk about, other than the time you woke up.

The world had come to a standstill, but not me. Even though I was stuck at home, I still kept going with my life. Things seemed great, even though COVID-19 was on the loose. I was happy that there was less work to complete for school. I had more time to sleep in. Overall, life was pretty easy. Life outside the home was hectic, though, and little did I know that things were about to get a bit crazy for me personally.

Soon, life went from dealing with the inconvenience of lockdown, into a total nightmare. Then, everything went down the drain.

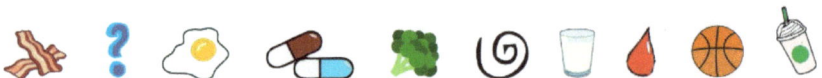

The Irregularity

At a time when the COVID-19 pandemic was taking many lives, surprisingly, it ushered me into a whole new discovery about my body. The pandemic itself never really scared me. I didn't go on playdates, sleepovers, or anything called social. But I like it that way, so COVID wasn't really a big deal. Then, I heard that lives were being lost. That totally freaked me out, and it scared the heebie-jeebies out of me.

I eventually calmed down. I had to. I had bigger problems to worry about. Looking back, I am grateful. Without the pandemic, I don't think I would have the awareness or knowledge I have right now.

At the same time that we were going into lockdown, I was having some irregularity in my period. I spotted but didn't actually have a full period for 2 months.

I had just turned twelve, so I didn't put too much thought into it. Irregular periods are typical. In the early onset of a period, this can be a normal part of the experience. I didn't feel or look different so I thought I was fine.

A little backstory:

I had my first period around 11 years old. According to studies, it is average. The youngest age to have your period is at 8, and the latest is usually 15. It could be later, depending on your genetics/background.

The changes I started to experience didn't really bother me until my mother called my attention to it. She was concerned. During this time I became more sluggish and very lazy. I didn't want to get up and I could and would sit in a chair for the whole day. This was not your typical "school is closed and there's nothing to do" kind of tired.

This was different. I definitely was not myself, and things felt very off.

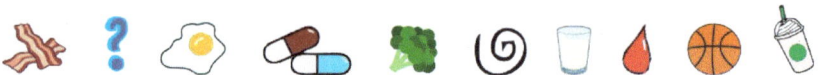

Alarming

By this time, my period had skipped 2 full months. Around April 27, 2020, my period finally started. I was happy that it finally did. I felt as if my period was holding a grudge against me and finally decided to let it go and talk to me again or in this case fill up a pad.

Little did I know, this would be the beginning of something I would never forget.

In prior months, my period would typically last 4-5 days. This time around was different. By May 15th, I was going on 2 whole weeks and 5 days of my period.

Two weeks and 5 days! Almost 3 weeks! That's the longest I've ever lasted.

This felt like an eternity that would never end.

I was still not bothered by this situation and I hoped it would remain that way for a while but it didn't. First of all, I was kinda excited that this was happening because in the process I lost about 5 pounds without exercising or going on a diet. Only 2 and half weeks! During COVID, when my activity level has decreased significantly, I still managed to lose a few pounds.

"This is awesome," I thought, at least for the time being. I wasn't bothered because I was too weak, too tired, void of strength to care what was happening. The other thought that seemed to flood my mind was, "I just hope I don't pass out."

That day, I used seven pads – the most I had ever used before.

This was alarming, something is definitely wrong! I became worried. So was my mom. What if the bleeding doesn't stop? What was going on with my body?

The doctor's office was closed due to COVID restrictions so I couldn't just waltz into my doctor's office with questions or even for a checkup. This was quite an eye-opener for me, showing me what Covid had done to the community.

At first, I didn't want to go to the doctor's office because I thought it would be embarrassing talking about blood, and how my period was irregular. I really don't like talking about myself and this situation was just pushing my limits. It was a relief that I wouldn't be seeing her in person.

The Prescription

The bleeding continued and I kept soaking up 7 pads each day. At this point, I was over it. I had had enough. Just end already!

At this point in my journey, I felt like I needed a break. It wasn't like I felt any pain. Most of the time I was lazy and just couldn't get out of bed or the couch. For someone who was an avid basketball player, a few weeks prior, this cannot be good!

Soon, I started feeling some numbness in my hands and feet. This never happened before, except when I sat on my hands or my feet stayed in the same place for a while.

This time was different. This time my hands were pale and drained of blood, it almost looked lifeless. My feet were very weak and I felt as if I could pass out any minute now. Then I started to feel very cold. I really was praying for a miracle because I really am starting to panic.

Two days went by, and my mom decided to consult with my pediatrician. Since the doctor couldn't see us in person she saw us on a video call.

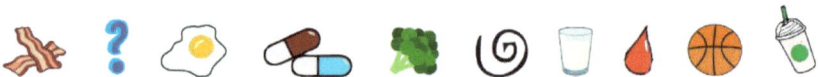

🥓 ❓ 🍳 💊 🥦 🌀 🥛 🩸 🏀 🥤

She asked me some questions. Remember, that I am twelve years old at the time.

Even though she was asking me these questions, she couldn't diagnose anything. Yet, she still recommended that I'd go on birth control. So imagine a 12-year-old girl, who isn't even a teenager yet, being told she would need to go on a birth control pill, for a medical reason that had yet to be diagnosed. Yeah, that's alarming!

That was a turn-off for me. I kinda thought I knew what birth control was. My initial thought was that birth control was for birthing-related issues. That didn't apply to me. I was confused.

After the meeting, I spoke with my mom because I was puzzled about why I would need birth control and what it would do for me. She then explained that a birth control pill would stop the bleeding, but the side effects were bloating, nausea, headaches, and other side effects. All the side effects really did disturb me.

"What type of doctor would want to put a twelve-year-old client through all of this?" This thought kept racing through my mind.

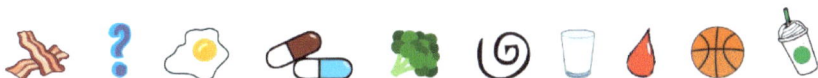

My mom reached out to a colleague who was a nurse and had grown daughters. Yea, she also reached out to my aunt who is a doctor. When my mom told me she asked her colleague and my aunt, I was struck with embarrassment. I didn't want anyone to know about what was going on with me. I wanted the doctors to know what was going on, and give me a remedy to make it go away before word got out.

Regardless, I was still hoping that they would have the answer.
Unfortunately, they all said something along the lines of a birth control pill. My mom's colleague shared a personal story of someone she knows who went on a birth control pill at the age of 16, with a similar bleeding situation. She mentioned that the heavy bleeding reduced, however it did not fully address the situation. At that moment, I felt that this was sorta comforting because I wasn't alone and the issue is more prevalent than I thought. Someone so close to home actually went through this. But then I caught myself thinking, wait a minute the problem didn't get resolved with the birth control pill. This is serious!

"The Inventory"

After the long outreach to friends and families, my mom reached a dead end. At this point, I really had no idea where to turn, except my bed, and just stay there for as long as this problem lasts. This whole situation was draining enough already, and the fact that no one knows what's wrong with me is draining every last inch of hope I have left.

Every opinion was pointing in the direction of a 12-year-old going on a birth control pill.
My mom told my sister and me to take an inventory of what we have been eating in the past few weeks of being homebound due to coronavirus.

Surprisingly we had been super healthy about what we ate. My mom would normally cook for us and she would switch up the order of what we ate in a week, so it wouldn't get boring. It never did.

We had a smoothie along with croissant, banana bread, or home-baked pastry for breakfast. Lunch was a sandwich, salad, beans, or homemade rice with chicken/fish. Dinner was similar to lunch but a small portion. Drinking water was a priority in our home. I drank some cranberry juice most of the time when I didn't feel like drinking water. Soda was occasional but I enjoyed it when I got the chance.

Mom suspected the increase in the use of whole milk with the smoothie, and possibly the berries was a factor in my extensive period. She really never had a proven reason for why milk and berries might be causing my problem, but advised me to stop it. We had to get an alternative (coconut milk). Coconut milk didn't have much of a taste to it, but my body was yearning for a solution. I still had to continue to travel down this curvy road.

I bled with no known reason; scared, confused, frail, and void of a solution.

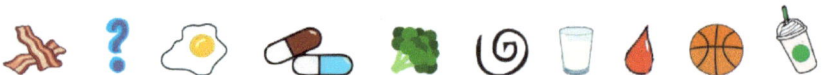

May 19th

By mid-May, the bleeding slowed down. It wasn't as heavy, but I was still at 7 pads for a day - not ideal. Three days had passed, and not much had changed. At this point, I was completely drained, physically and mentally.

Just when I thought things couldn't get much worse, I found myself in the emergency room. There was numbness in my fingers and toes. I was dizzy.

On the way to the hospital, all sorts of things were going through my mind.

"Will they have any answers?
Would my life be like this forever?
Am I slowly dying?"

The doctors ran all kinds of tests and gave me IV fluids. The doctor said my hemoglobin had dropped to 9.4. Hemoglobin, I learned, is a protein in your red blood cells that carries oxygen to your body's organs and tissues and transports carbon dioxide from your organs and tissues back to your lungs. If a hemoglobin test reveals that your hemoglobin level is lower than normal, it means you have a low red blood cell count (anemia). (Mayo Clinic)"

At this point, my hemoglobin wasn't low enough to have a blood transfusion. It needed to drop to 7 or below for that. That was a relief because I don't want anything to do with needles, blood, or anything hospital related

To receive a blood transfusion, it can be complicated. You need to get a matching blood type. Do I even know my blood type? Is there my blood type in the hospital? My mind couldn't stop racing with questions. My poor mother gently helped calm my mind down, by telling me the blood transfusion is for the doctors to worry about.

 Either way, they sent me home at this point. Still no reason for what was going on.

I felt frustrated. The doctors had no answers. Nobody knew what was happening. I knew they were trying their best, but I just want someone, even something to be the solution. I wanted answers. I felt like I was being tipped over the edge and I didn't like it.

I had to take a deep breath and try to relax, and find patience. There was nothing that could be done, so I returned home with the plan to see a specialist for my hormone levels.

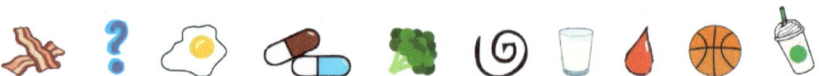

Enzymes

When I got home from the emergency room, mom and I consulted with a nutritionist, who took an inventory of my meals, just like my mom previously did. Even though the doctors didn't recommend a nutritionist, my mom thought it would be a good idea.

Going into the meeting with her, I wasn't getting my hopes up too high. I didn't want my hopes to be shattered. I didn't want to be crushed all over again and I had heard too much bad news and seen too many dead ends as it was already.

She noted that I had a relatively balanced meal plan. She also noticed one other thing. My food intake didn't include foods that are rich in fat and fiber. She asked if I didn't like fatty foods and food rich in fiber, or if I even knew what those were. Then she asked if I liked the following foods: bacon or eggs.

I told her I hated eating those foods. I explained to her that I used to love bacon, but along the way I hated it. It didn't taste right or smell right to me. I also explained to her that I've always hated the look and smell of eggs. I didn't mind the taste of the white part of a boiled egg, though, since it had no taste. It wouldn't be my first choice, though. Then I explained that every time I ate bacon my stomachs started to hurt really bad to the point that I would need to bend over or lie on the ground.

The nutritionist said I have a smart body because my body knows those foods are difficult for me to digest. As a result, I subconsciously have a dislike for it. She recommended I use an enzyme to digest the fat that my body had been avoiding silently. The enzyme was a pill that I took. It was kinda' big to me, and I really tried to avoid pills since they are very hard for me to swallow.

The enzyme would assist my body in breaking down the fat, making it easier for me to eat fatty foods without dealing with excruciating pain. The nutritionist advised that if fatty foods like bacon and egg yolk continue to hurt my stomach/body, then I should find other alternative foods to provide the fat I need.

She explained since I'm in puberty and my body needs those foods, it is slowly weighing on my overall health. She asked if I felt pain or discomfort on the left side of my body, which I confirmed to her was accurate. She also asked how my sleep routine was lately. I told her I have been having

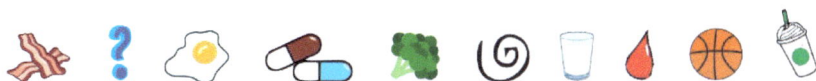

interrupted sleep lately (waking up in the middle of the night).

She confirmed to me that my overall system is under stress due to the nutritional deprivation from the fat and fiber which is in turn affecting my endocrine system. The endocrine system is the collection of glands that produce hormones that regulate metabolism, reproduction, sleep, mood, amongst other things. I am beginning to have a whoa moment. This all makes sense!
A change in diet was the result of the consultation with the nutritionist. In a matter of days, the enzyme changed the number of pads I had to use. I was down to 5 pads daily.
Even though I didn't have my full energy back I was starting to have hope. I was on my way to feeling better, or so I thought.

The Setback

You know how some people have cheat days? A cheat day is when someone eats something that they are not supposed to eat, either because they're on a diet, or because it's bad for them. Well, I don't cheat days. I never needed them before this phase of my life. I always had the privilege of eating whatever I wanted. My mom would just remind me that I'm eating too much in a short period. If I had a cheat day I'd probably eat cookies since I'm known as the Cookie Monster. Also because I love cookies.

Sadly, a trip to Target with my mother and sister set me back on my journey to wellness.
I spotted a Starbucks within the Target store, and it felt like the seasonal drink, S'mores, was calling my name. We went to Starbucks and I decided to order it. Not wanting to consume whole milk, I thought that replacing whole milk with coconut milk would make everything okay.
Boy! Was I wrong? S'mores had chocolate, whipped cream, chocolate syrup and all of it contained dairy and none of which was friendly to my body.

I didn't even finish half of the drink! Within a few minutes, though, I noticed I wasn't feeling so good.

Then, I realized, I started to bleed again with clots. They were twice the size of a quarter, and there were multiple of them.

It was at that moment, I realized, it was time to listen to my body. If I didn't, my life would never be the same. If I don't take control and monitor what I eat, then I would end up having a blood transfusion and a lifelong problem.

I have a message to share with the world at large. My misery from drinking the S'mores drink lasted for 3 days. I couldn't believe it. I was finally on the right track to being normal again and a small drink shattered my dreams. I was devastated.

If only I had thought a little harder I would have caught all the other ingredients with dairy in it. I had to go to the ER again so they could make sure my hemoglobin hadn't dropped below the normal range. The doctor said that my hemoglobin had dropped to 8.4 and that if it drops to 7.0 I would need a blood transfusion. The thought of having a blood transfusion was already out there but now that I knew that I was 1.4 blood levels from having a blood transfusion.

I became even more apprehensive. The doctor at the ER recommended that I see a hormone specialist as it appeared I was showing early signs of endometriosis. He mentioned that a visit to the hormone specialist will help rule out endometriosis even though he did say that it's a diagnosis that can not be made due to my age.

A follow-up call was made to my nutritionist who advised that I get coconut water to replenish the lost fluid and keep my electrolytes up.
A visit was scheduled to the hormone specialist doctor which took about a week. I explained to the doctor my symptoms and how I've managed them so far. She expressed that this is quite unusual with the period going on for such a long time. At this point, it had been 29 days!

She took necessary blood work and advised that it could be early signs of endometriosis, but no formal diagnosis can be made at this age. It was at that moment that my mom and I agreed that we will aggressively pursue the nutritional measures we have been following.

I had multiple questions like what is endometriosis? Can endometriosis kill you? Is endometriosis painful? At this point, I was so confused because I had no idea what

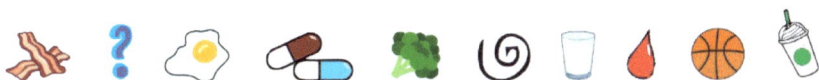

endometriosis was and I didn't want to know. I was too scared of what was to come.

A few articles I read affirmed the doctor's position on me being too young to be diagnosed with endometriosis.

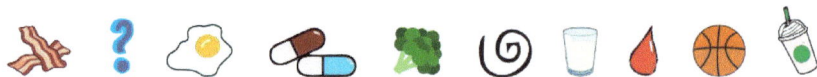

The Normalcy

After meeting with the hormone specialist, she listened to me tell me what led to the referral from the ER visit. She did blood work on me and advised that no formal diagnosis can be made yet. The result of the blood work doesn't come in for another couple of days.

She mentioned that I might have to use a birth control pill even though I'm quite young for it. I felt defeated hearing this doctor say the same thing as the others. This cannot be the solution to my problem. I must do something fast! I had to revamp my eating, drinking, and activity level completely. I changed my eating habits and stayed away from dairy completely until I was well regulated. I followed my diet strictly. I stayed away from dairy and eggs (the yolk).

 I also stayed away from foods with low or no fat. I avoided processed sugar. I stayed away from anything with pork and berries. The berries made me cramp really badly and the pork made me nauseous. The foods that I avoided did help me in the long run and my stomachs started to feel a lot better. As you may be thinking, what food did I eat? Well, I loaded up on some new foods like:

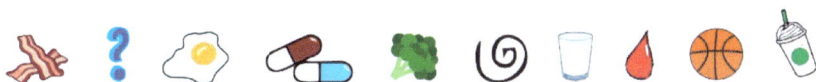

Protein: banana nut bread, smoothie
(mango/pineapple/banana/acai),
Chicken/Hamburger sandwich, Chicken with salad,
turkey, caesar wrap, beans, crab, salmon

Fat/Fiber: coconut milk, pear, butter, walnuts,
shredded carrot, fruit salad
(soul bowl), walnuts, pineapple

Vegetable: pepper, onions, broccoli, salad, kale,
spinach

Carbohydrate: croissant, cereal, yam, bread, rice,
noodles, potato fries, noodles, potato fries, corn,
plantain

Drink: water, cranberry, fruit juice

By June 2nd, I was down to 3 - 4 pads a day. I
continued with my strict diet and the use of my
nutritional enzymes. I made routine visits to my
nutritionist until she advised me to stop the
prescribed enzymes.

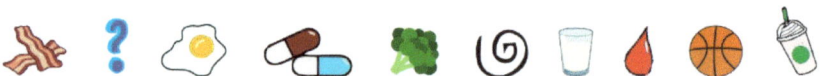

Fast forward to June 12th my period finally stopped. It was indeed a celebration at my house and for me! I thought this day would never come. I had embedded myself into a lot of reading and research about my crisis, and the onset of endometriosis. The stories I read were not quite promising. There was literature and the account of others that highlighted this as a hereditary, feminine issue with no known cause. I knew I didn't want to fit into these statistics.

I'm an athlete. I live a very active lifestyle, and this made it all vanish! I couldn't let that happen because basketball is what I look forward to every year. I love the fact that I can run and dribble at the same time, and have a clock still running, waiting for someone to make that first shot. My life without basketball is not a life at all. I can not afford to let endometriosis take over my life when I know I can do something.

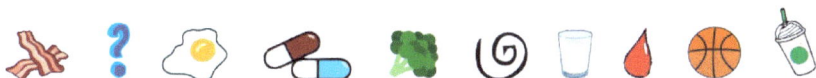

The 7 Takeaways

- Endometriosis can have an early onset as young as 11 years old.
- If someone in your family has endometriosis you are 7-10 times likely to have it than someone without a family history of it.
- A well-planned diet by a nutritionist can help alleviate the early onset of endometriosis. An early planned diet regimen will save you years of pain and repeated doctor's visits.
- Young adults are more resilient.
- Know your body; diet is key to healthy womanhood.

- Be smart with your body; see a nutritionist; get a food inventory.

- No girl or woman should live in pain

Some General Notes for the Reader

Endometriosis is a disorder in which tissue that normally lines the uterus grows outside the uterus. With endometriosis, the tissue can be found on the ovaries, fallopian tubes, or intestines. The most common symptoms are pain and menstrual irregularities. Effective treatments, such as hormones and excision surgery, are available.

In my story, I talk a lot about diets and watching what you eat. Endometriosis is not a dietary concern, it is an actual disorder. The reason why I talk a lot about watching what you eat is that that is what got me through these tough times. I really had to sit back and see what could be doing this to me. I'm not saying that watching your diet is the cure; I'm just saying that it can help in the long run.

The symptoms of endometriosis are irregular periods and pain. During my journey, I did deal with cramps that made me lean forward (hunch over) and grab my stomach. The cramps were more of a discomfort. I do consider myself as someone with high pain tolerance. It takes a lot for me to feel a painful sensation.

In my family, a few people do have endometriosis, like my great aunt, and my grandmother, and a few

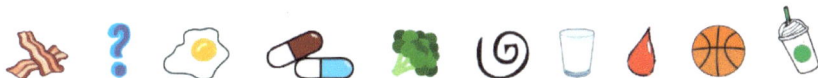

of my cousins. I think that's where I got it. Some of them had surgery which did help them. Understanding your body can be hard but there are ways for you to get close and in touch with what your body may be trying to say to you. First of all, you need to keep track of the foods and drinks, and how you feel after you consume them.

Another thing you can do is to see the outcomes of what happens when you are active or vice versa. Basically, just list down what a daily routine might look like for you and try to narrow down what things hurt you and what things benefit your body.

During this time, when my nutritional intake was under scrutiny, my nutritionist mentioned that I am showing the beginning stages of endometriosis. Endometriosis is unfortunately not diagnosed until the '20s or '30s, however, teenagers and young adults experience symptoms during adolescence. My nutritionist described my body as being smart to have reacted in the way it did, so I can take measures to prevent full onset of endometriosis.

Lastly, I would like to share the final takeaway that I like to leave with the readers. When I started my book I was afraid and had moments I thought there was no need to write this book. As I said before,

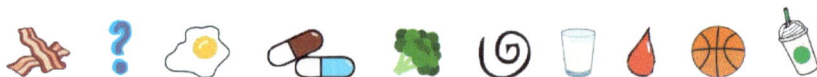

talking about your period is awkward and can sometimes be uncomfortable.

But putting all my thoughts on paper has actually turned out to be very gratifying. Having really personal conversations can be difficult, but you have to do it if it can make a difference. Getting to know my body and what it likes and dislikes is a totally new adventure for me. Listening to your body may be challenging but totally rewarding.

Thank You

Writing this book is harder than I thought, and more rewarding than I could have ever imagined.

None of this would have been possible without my loving mom, Tosin. She told me my story will help someone out there.

Thank you, my little sister, Esther, for always going on this nutritional path with me. You choose to not eat the foods that were only hurtful to me. You say, "We are in this together."

Thanks to my dad, Moses, for always being "Doctor Dad."

I'm eternally grateful to my two nutritionists, Dr. Penny Goldstein and Drema, you both empowered me to know my body. I truly had no idea what was happening to my young body. You both provided me with the knowledge I have now and will forever share.

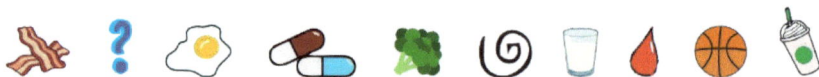

About the Author

Bavaria G. is a first-time author. Bavaria is a daughter, sister, and friend.

She lives an active life as an athlete for 7 years and counting.

Besides being athletic, Bavaria loves to do other things like sewing, origami, and of course writing.

Bavaria has a strong passion for writing which helped motivate her to write this book. Sharing this story has meant so much to her, and she is ready to do so much more with her writing career.

www.ingramcontent.com/pod-product-compliance
Lightning Source LLC
Chambersburg PA
CBHW041220270326
41931CB00005B/119